Smal

Put The Odds In Your Favor!
1st Edition - Print - 2017

ISBN-10: 0-9967053-3-3
ISBN-13: 978-0-9967053-3-2

Content	**Design & Layout**	**Editors**
Michelle Robin	Zachary Cole,	Rebecca Korphage
Shelly Murray	Chisik Studio	Kayti Doolittle

For information, address Michelle Robin, D.C.
7410 Switzer, Shawnee Mission, KS 66203
or e-mail: mrobin@drmichellerobin.com

Disclaimer: No book, including this one, can replace the services of
a qualified physician or other health-care professional. If problems
appear or persist, the reader should consult with a well-chosen
physician, health-care or mental-health professional. Accordingly,
the author/creator expressly disclaim any liability, loss, damage
or injury caused by the contents of this book.

While I never recommend anything that I don't use and love myself,
I am an affiliate for some products and services listed in this book
and may be compensated if you purchase them through the links
provided in the online End Notes for this book, or via the Shop on
my website. I want to be transparent, because your trust means
everything to me, and I'll never compromise that.

TABLE OF CONTENTS

ACCESS ONLINE END NOTES

This book is also offered as an interactive ebook full of links to podcast interviews, videos, and resources that relate to the content in each section throughout the book. We've created a special web page, called End Notes, for you to access that same content.

You can find it at: www.drmichellerobin.com/scbs-online-end-notes

There you'll find related online content that enriches and further explores what you read in this book. It is organized by the same chapter titles to make it easy to navigate. If you're interested in getting the ebook version of this printed book you can download it at www.quadrantsofwellbeing.com.

INTRODUCTION

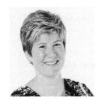 In 2017 I am celebrating 25 years guiding people on their wellness journeys. That's half my life! I feel grateful every day that I get to help people make those small changes that ultimately shift their whole lives. I love helping them put the odds in their favor and celebrate their wins along the way.

Twenty-five years ago my chiropractic practice was just me seeing clients one-on-one. I had a vision to grow into an integrative wellness center which became Your Wellness Connection℠ (YWC). YWC has now been in its current custom built home for 15 years. The last 10 years YWC has grown and changed to meet the needs of clients while being right-sized for the changes in my life, allowing me to serve you in different ways – as a speaker, author, podcaster, and by creating courses and programs. My drive has always been to inspire you to connect with your body-mind-spirit, to learn how and take actions that will put the odds of health and wellness in your favor.

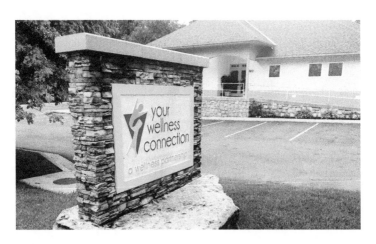

Wellbeing doesn't just happen. It takes consistent, mindful effort to gain, maintain, or regain. We all start where we are. You may be a triathlete whose health and fitness is always front and center, and you're looking for new ways to maintain your wellbeing. You may be rather healthy, near your ideal weight or a bit overweight, but you're starting to feel the changes in energy, flexibility, and resilience that come with age, so you're seeking a change. You may be dealing with a chronic illness, injury, or obesity, and you're searching for simple changes you can start making today to create a different future. Or you may be in perfect health and want to keep it that way.

No matter where you are on the wellbeing spectrum, start with gratitude. Be grateful for the body you currently have. Your body is doing the best it can right now to care for you. As you honor your body, be mindful of where you can make small changes to give yourself what you need to move more towards health and wellness, continuing to put the odds in your favor.

As you are on your wellness journey, I encourage you to always listen to your body and work on creating a harmonious plan. This plan should work for you and your individual needs. If you go to the online End Notes (see page 1 of this book for instructions) for this book you'll find a link to the Body Talk Quiz. The questions help identify if major systems in your body are under stress. Your results from Body Talk may be the beginnings of a plan. It's one way to know where to start to improve your health and wellbeing.

This book is filled with many tips for creating your wellness plan. Try to incorporate some of the healthy habits mentioned and consider utilizing some of the resources listed in the back of the book.

Hugs,

Michelle Robin

PS - This book holds a lot of helpful and healthful power for such a small package. My goal is to get this in the hands of 1 Million people.

Please send your friends to www.quadrantsofwellbeing.com where they can download a free copy of the ebook version. Thank you!

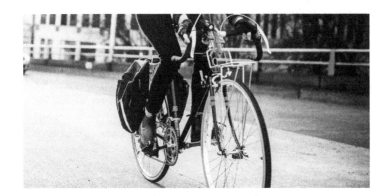

ODDS IN MY FAVOR

Your current state of wellbeing is not to be taken for granted. It can be compromised in an instant. I know because it happened to me.

In June of 2015 I was on an early morning bike ride, training for a sprint triathlon, when I was clipped by a car. The result was ten fractures in my pelvis, hip, elbow, and thumb. I was laid up and unable to practice chiropractic for many months. The experience thoroughly tested my mind, body and spirit wellbeing.

I've learned many lessons from that time and have since. I want to share a few with you here to put you in the right frame of mind as you read this book and take action. If I had not spent the previous decade plus putting the odds in my favor for wellbeing, I very likely could have lost my business, my livelihood, my health, and much of my heart as a result of the accident.

Whether it is an accident, a chronic disease, a death in the family, the loss of a relationship, or a sudden illness, the work you do now will serve you as you heal, recover, and move forward.

FIVE TIPS FOR PUTTING THE ODDS IN YOUR FAVOR

1. **Heal your heart.** In my early 30's I participated in The Hoffman Process. Those seven days changed my life forever. During that week, I learned to forgive, let go and change the script that had been playing in my mind for years. Healing my heart helped me build a successful practice, maintain a loving relationship with my friends and family and helped me stay strong after my accident. Wellness, health and happiness all starts with matters of the heart.

2. **Know your why.** Is it being there for your children, playing with grandchildren, being able to be active, or being healthy enough to live out your purpose? Regardless of your motivation, it is always easier to stay on the path of wellbeing if you're clear about where you're going and your why.

3. **Take consistent action.** Wellbeing is not something you can just buy in bulk at Costco when you need it. It is something you build day by day over time. That's why I believe in small changes. They're easier to make, do consistently, and fully integrate into your life. One small change can create a big shift in your wellbeing. Many small changes over time create a vibrant life. But you have to take action.

4. **Find your tribe.** Jim Rohn once famously said that we are the average of the five people we spend the most time with...whether we like it or not the people around us can affect our mood, our habits and even our self-esteem. So the question is do you have a tribe that supports the life you want to live? They are the like-minded people with whom you surround yourself. They encourage and support you along the way. As you build your tribe, invite them to join you on this venture.

5. **Celebrate the wins.** As I was healing and recovering from the accident there were days it took everything out of me just to move across the room. I learned to celebrate every tiny success. They compound to create huge wins in your wellness journey.

Others – government, insurance companies, and health care providers - will continue to volley back and forth about how to make healthcare affordable. The reality is that it doesn't have to be up to them. True affordability starts with us, each taking responsibility for our wellbeing. The ideas and resources you'll find in the pages that follow will help you put the odds in your favor for a healthy and well life...if you take action. It's up to you. You can do it!

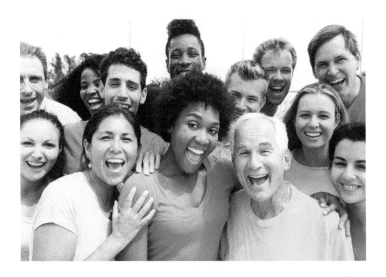

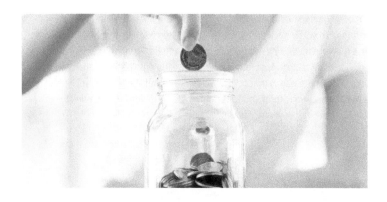

WELLNESS CREDITS AND DEBITS

Wellness is cumulative. It is like a bank account with credits, debits and compounding interest. Each choice, each action, each thought either adds to your mind-body-spirit wellbeing or subtracts from it. The next choice, action or thought either credits your wellness account or debits it. And the next.

What is your overall account at the end of the day?

If we're talking about your actual bank account, the more you add to it the more capable you are of spending something for a treat or handling a major expense without going broke. The same is true for your health and wellness account. The more you build up your mental, emotional, spiritual, and physical wellbeing, the more you have to spend. You will have the energy to do everything you want, the capacity to love and be loved, a stronger faith, or the ability to heal quickly and resist illness. Wealth in wellness affords you the internal resources for both the joys in life and the difficulties.

All too often we go, go, go, pushing ourselves, stretching our limits, and debiting our health accounts to the point that we get tapped out. Then someone or something happens that requires our time, energy and focus, and the only way we can give it is to tap our reserves. The problem is that if we constantly dip into our savings (energy reserves) one day there is little left when we actually need it, or worse yet, we are completely drained. This is when people have a major health event, crash, and break down. It is like living paycheck to paycheck with mounting debt and suddenly the income disappears. Some recover quickly from the crisis; others aren't so lucky and declare bankruptcy. They'll get back on their feet eventually, but it will take time. Keep your coffers full by making healthy choices, crediting your account. The more you slowly add to your wellness account, the more you are able to draw from it to live a vibrant life.

Positive actions and thoughts that credit your wellness account accumulate, and with compounding interest. Today, you may only be able to walk to the end of your street and back. But if you walked that short distance every day, by the end of the month you would likely be circling the block twice. When you break down your overall goals into manageable chunks you will feel the accumulation of health. As you begin to add more healthy choices while maintaining the habits you've already created, it is as if you are gaining the compounding interest of health. However the flip side is true as well. If you don't invest in your health now you miss out on the accumulating affects. The time will come when you need that health wealth, and it won't be there; instead you'll be facing a big bill with no resources to pay. The good news...you can always start today.

I practice client care in a holistic manner considering and addressing the Quadrants of Wellbeing. As you learn about each quadrant I share with you credits you can make to your whole body health account. As you increase your credits you help assure a healthy, positive balance. However too many debits will only lead to a negative bottom line and wellness bankruptcy. Think about how you may be currently crediting or bankrupting that part of your wellbeing, as we explore each quadrant. Keep in mind how everything you think and do credits or debits your wellbeing. Take it day by day, choice by choice, one small change at a time.

QUADRANTS OF WELLBEING

We all know people who exercise a lot, but aren't healthy, people who are vegan, but aren't healthy, and people who meditate or pray regularly who aren't healthy.

Being healthy and well takes more than being diligent in one area of wellness. It requires attentiveness to your whole person – body, mind and spirit. The Quadrants of Wellbeing provide a framework for supporting whole being wellness.

MECHANICAL
Physical Body

CHEMICAL
What We Put In and On Our Body

ENERGY
Life Force

- Psychospiritual
- Mechanical
- Chemical
- Energy

Psychospiritual: The mind and spirit influence the body in ways that are undeniable and not fully understood. Emotional and spiritual blocks can stress the body creating pain and dysfunction.

TIPS FOR **PSYCHOSPIRITUAL WELLNESS** *(Mental/Emotional Awareness)*
1. Be mindful of every moment.
2. Do something you love every day.
3. Think about 10 reasons you are grateful for your body.
4. Say no...
5. Treat yourself with as much compassion as you would a friend.

Mechanical: The physical body - muscles, ligaments, bones, tissue - is remarkable. It's meant to move while being flexible and strong.

TIPS FOR **MECHANICAL WELLNESS** *(Physical Body)*

1. Have monthly check-ups with your Chiropractor; get adjusted, if necessary.
2. Improve your sleep posture - by using a pillow with proper neck support. Avoid sleeping on your stomach or with your arms overhead.
3. Be active! Move! Take 8,000-10,000 steps per day. When you are at work use the stairs. When you are at the grocery store or parking at an event park farther from the door.
4. Use a headset while talking on the phone.
5. Improve your posture - If you sit in a chair at work that is not ergonomically designed, add a small pillow behind your lower back for lumbar support.

Chemical: Our chemistry is influenced by what we eat, drink, breathe, think, put on our skin, and how we process stress.

TIPS FOR **CHEMICAL WELLNESS** *(What We Put In And On Our Body)*

1. Make vegetables 50% of your food consumption. You can consume vegetables raw, cooked, steamed, as juice, or in a smoothie.
2. Drink an 8 oz. glass of water and eat breakfast before you drink coffee.
3. Include a high quality fat with every meal.
4. Eat away from your desk and the TV.
5. Chew your food 20-30 times per bite.

Energetic: The life-energy that courses through your body is influenced by external environments and energy sources.

TIPS FOR **ENERGETIC WELLNESS** *(Life Force)*

1. Take five deep breaths upon waking and before going to sleep. Make sure to take deep breaths when you are in stressful situations too.
2. Take one hour a day away from technology.
3. Take a hot shower, bath or sauna session before bed and visualize letting go of the energy from the day.
4. Create a regular sleep routine.
5. Use technology like BrainTap® to relax your mind and reduce stress.

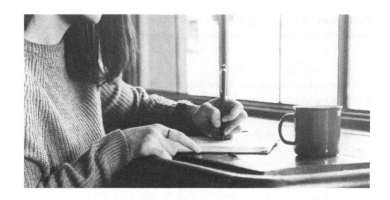

TOP 12 SMALL CHANGES

---

1. Email or text three things you are grateful for today to friends or family; or write them down in a gratitude journal.

2. Put yourself on your calendar. Spend 30 to 60 minutes planning your wellbeing for the week. Plan and schedule your meals, exercise, family time and self-care. Make yourself a priority and try to give yourself at least 2 hours of alone time a week.

3. Start your day with water. If you do not have a citrus sensitivity then add a lemon to your water. Drink 1/2 your body weight in ounces. (If you weigh 150 lbs., drink 75 oz. of water.)

4. Try fasting. Drink bone broth for 24 hours. To make fasting easier start your morning with breakfast and eat lunch. Then drink bone broth for dinner. Continue your bone broth for breakfast and lunch the next day. Then you can eat a salad for dinner. If you have health challenges consult a doctor before fasting.

5. Understand your genetics so you know what the future may hold, health-wise, and you can put the odds in your favor, learning what you can do to reverse, prevent, or delay issues.

6. Make sure to get 7 to 9 hours of sleep a night.

7. Eat your veggies.

8. Listen to your body, mind and spirit daily. When you find yourself agitated, bloated or not sleeping play private eye and figure out why! These changes are your body talking to you. Listen.

9. Celebrate yourself and others. At the end of each day write down one action or moment you are proud of. Celebrate your journey, process and little or big wins.

10. Have dinner with your significant other or someone in your "tribe" at least once a week, just the two of you. Let them dominate the conversation and try not to talk about work. Listen. Be present.

11. Carve out ten uninterrupted minutes every day for your children or your furry family members. In those 10-minutes make sure to listen to them. Sometimes the best way to love someone is to listen to what they say.

12. Start your day with prayer, meditation or an affirmation. End your day with gratitude.

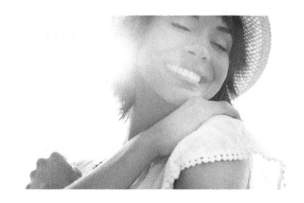

SELF-COMPASSION

"The curious paradox is that when I accept myself just as I am, then I can change." - **Carl Rogers**

THE POWER OF SELF-COMPASSION

Stress. Heartbreak. Failure. We all experience it. Maybe you missed a deadline, or ate a bag of chips when you were supposed to be on a diet because you had a fight with your spouse. Maybe your child is struggling in school, or you lost your job and your savings is dwindling. In these stressful moments it is easy to get lost in your own mind, consumed with a constant current of repetitive negative thoughts. In these moments, what you need more than anything is self-compassion.

WHAT IS SELF-COMPASSION?

Self-compassion is a willingness to look at yourself and your perceived shortcomings with kindness and empathy. Dr. Kristin Neff, a self-compassion expert and researcher, explains that self-compassion involves acting the same way towards yourself as you would a friend. Neff explains when you practice self-compassion in a stressful or trying moment, you don't ignore your pain. Instead you tell yourself: *"This is really difficult right now. How can I comfort and care for myself in this moment?"*

I know for me personally, I had to practice a lot of self-compassion after my accident in 2015. Due to the extent of my injuries and the trauma to my nervous system, it was six months before I could fully walk again. People who know me well, know how difficult staying still was for me. I was used to being the doctor not the patient. If I had not practiced self-compassion during my healing journey I am not sure I would be where I am today.

Today, I am a better chiropractor, friend and partner than I have ever been because I understand healing in a way I never did before. Whether you are trying to quit smoking, trying to release those stubborn ten pounds or experiencing a tremendous loss, self-compassion is the key. It is the secret to overcoming any obstacle we encounter in our lifetime.

THE SCIENCE OF SELF-COMPASSION

Don't just take my word for it. Research is now showing how cultivating self-compassion can change us for the better.

According to Dr. Neff's research, practicing self-compassion can...
- Lead to higher levels of personal wellbeing
- Reduce chronic stress
- Ease depression and anxiety
- Improve interpersonal relationships
- Enhance patience, generosity and gratitude
- Boost hormones like oxytocin and cortisol

ARE YOU SELF COMPASSIONATE OR SELF-CRITICAL?

We are taught to be problem solvers. In many ways these skills keep us safe and help us progress in our relationships, school, business and life. They help us survive. The problem arrives when we get stuck in negative thought patterns such as:

"I will never be enough."
"I always give up on diets."
"I failed in my last job. What's the point?"

These thoughts can lead to shame, depression and really they keep us from thriving. If you are wondering if you are too hard on yourself, take Dr. Kristin Neff's online self-compassion quiz, which you can find at www.self-compassion.org.

SELF-COMPASSION AND BODY IMAGE

Did you know...
- 50% of 3 to 6 year olds worry about being fat?
- Over 50% of females between the ages of 18 to 25 would prefer to be run over by a truck than be fat.
- Concern about the body and eating problems is the number one issue for girls and women aged 11 to 80 years–if not about themselves then about their daughters and granddaughters.

I encountered these staggering statistics when I spoke with Dr. Laura Eickman the founder of REbeL. REbeL is a student-driven education program designed to address body image issues and disordered eating.

What I realized after meeting Dr. Eickman is that it isn't just young women that suffer from negative body image. Men and women of all ages are caught in a cycle of negative self-talk about their bodies. I also realized that practicing self-compassion is essential as we age, since our bodies change in appearance and physical ability. Self-compassion is a lifelong practice.

Psychotherapist and author of *The Self-Compassion Diet,* Jean Fain, has a list of questions you can ask yourself if you think you might be too self-critical. Ask yourself the questions below. If you answer yes to two or more, you may want to try incorporating more self-compassion into your every day life.

1. Do you hate looking at photos of yourself?
2. Do you hate shopping for clothes?
3. Can stepping on the scale ruin your day?
4. Does seeing yourself naked upset you?

5. Does eating a full meal stress you out?
6. Do you feel badly about your body when you see models and celebrities?
7. Do you avoid bathing suits and revealing clothes?
8. Does socializing with attractive people make you feel self-conscious?

Questions sourced from The Self-Compassion Diet, Jean Fain.

HOW TO PRACTICE SELF-COMPASSION

The truth is, without self-compassion it can be really hard to sustain a healthy diet or exercise. Our potential success, health and happiness all starts with our heart.

The good news is practicing self-compassion isn't complicated.

Here are a few strategies you can try to deepen or create a self-compassion practice.

1. Treat yourself like you would your best friend. In moments of pain and stress be gentle and kind.

2. Say YES to yourself. Listen to your body and your needs. Give your body what it needs and don't judge it.

3. Give yourself a hug! Or you can even comfort yourself by putting your hands over your heart. The gesture doesn't really matter as long as it is comforting to you.

4. Make sure to watch your language and how you speak to yourself. Let go of self-judgment. If you are beating yourself up for messing up a diet or not exercising today, let it go.

5. Read compassionate affirmations daily. I have loved reading *I Declare* by Joel Osteen every day. Choose what speaks to your heart.

6. Listen to your body. What does it need? I know my body often thrives when I start my day with a green smoothie. What makes your body thrive today?

7. Practice a guided Loving Kindness Meditation.

8. I always wear my favorite socks. Notes to Self Socks® contain affirmations like *I am Thankful, I am Kind and I am Strong.*

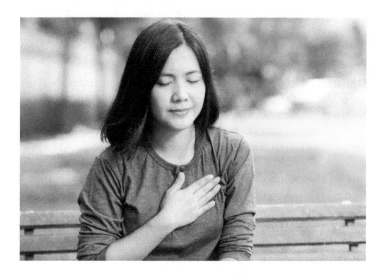

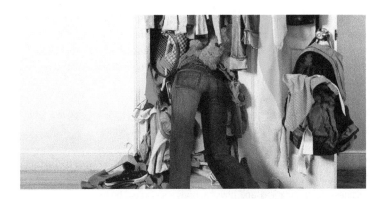

FREE YOUR SPACE

When we think of clutter we often think about stuff. Yet, clutter isn't just about the physical accumulation of things, or stuff out of place. Many of us live with massive amounts of clutter and don't even know it.

CLUTTER HAS MANY FORMS

- The old instruction manuals, broken pens and unopened mail we stuff in our junk drawer just in case
- The ever-growing debt on our credit card
- Our chaotic closet exploding with unworn clothes
- The negative words we replay in our mind over and over
- Gossip
- The bad memories, regrets, or anger we hold onto for far too long
- An over-scheduled life and unchecked busyness
- Our inbox, overrun with emails, many of which we never read
- The frozen pizza you had for dinner last night, and all the other unhealthy food and beverages you consume

Most of us have no idea how much clutter affects us. It isn't until we start clearing it out that we realize how much better we feel without it; which is how I felt when I right-sized my life in 2013. I wrote several blogs about it and the lessons and revelations through the process of right-sizing. Check the online End Notes for links.

For me, it wasn't about becoming a minimalist. It wasn't about living in a tiny house, getting rid of all my books or never eating french fries.

It was about letting go of the stuff, practices, and thought patterns that didn't lift my soul. It was about decluttering and freeing my spaces - my home, business, calendar, mind, and physical body - so I could be my best, most joyful self. **For me, it was about living intentionally.**

I wanted to trade stuff for health, for love, for time, and for a life that didn't revolve around compulsory consumption, and other people's definitions of success.

IF YOU WANT TO EXPERIMENT WITH DECLUTTERING, HERE ARE 6 SIMPLE WAYS YOU CAN START TO FREE YOUR SPACE TODAY

1. **Listen to my podcast with the lovely Courtney Carver.** Courtney is the founder of the blog, *Be More with Less.* She writes about the power of living a simple clutter-free life and how it has personally transformed her health. You can find the link in the online End Notes.

2. **Surround yourself with happiness.** Everything is energy. And everything has and holds energy. How are the objects, people, and foods you eat making you feel? If you have objects that give you the slightest pang of sadness, guilt, frustration, anger, or hurt let them go. Depending on what it is, you can sell it, donate it, offer it up to friends and family who might want it (especially heirlooms), or throw it away. You can also let people go by gently disconnecting from them. This is actually a practice of self-compassion! Watch as your energy shifts.

3. **Get a little inspiration or perspective before you start decluttering.** Watch, *Minimalism, A Documentary About Important Things.* Courtney Carver is

sharing her story in this film as well. Also check out the documentary *May I Be Frank,* where my friend, Frank Ferrante, declutters his life from a completely different perspective.

4. **Pick one processed food item that you regularly consume and commit to eliminating it from your diet for one week.** Journal about how you feel. If you add it back in later, pay attention to how it makes you feel after not having it for a while.

5. **Not ready to clean out your closet? Simply take the clothes you have not been wearing and place them in another closet.** If you don't wear them for 6-months, if you don't even notice they are gone, then you will know, it's time to let them go. (Remember, to donate them! That sweater you never wear might make another person feel beautiful.)

6. **Last but not least, practice gratitude.** Sometimes we get stuck in unhealthy patterns. We focus on the love our parents never gave us, and fail to see the love right in front of us. We look at our lives and see lack, instead of all the love, beauty and possibility. Sit down today and write a very specific list of five things you are grateful to have in your life. Do this daily.

Now, if after these six steps you still feel overwhelmed and under-inspired, then I invite you to check out my online program, *21 Days to Free Your Space.* Be prepared to clear your spaces: environments, body, heart and mind. You can find it in the Shop at my website, www.drmichellerobin.com.

POSITIVE THOUGHTS

Words matter. They can tear down or build up. They can create woe or inspiration and hope. This is true for what you read, listen to, or say to yourself or others. Choose to fill your mind, spirit, and voice with uplifting words. I've shared some of my favorite quotes below.

"The groundwork of all happiness is good health."
– Leigh Hunt

"No matter how much I get done, or is left undone,
at the end of the day, I AM ENOUGH."
– Brene Brown

"If you can't fly, then run, if you can't run, then walk, if you can't walk, then
crawl, but whatever you do, you have to keep moving forward."
– Martin Luther King Jr.

"Feeling gratitude and not expressing it is like
wrapping a present and not giving it."
– William Arthur Ward

"Kindness is a language which the deaf and the blind can read."
– Mark Twain

"The journey of a thousand miles begins with a single step."
– Lao Tzu

"The first wealth is health."
– Ralph Waldo Emerson

"Take care of your body. It's the only place you live."
– Jim Rohn

"The planet does not need more 'successful people.' The planet desperately
needs more peacemakers, healers, restorers, storytellers and lovers of all kinds."
– Dalai Lama

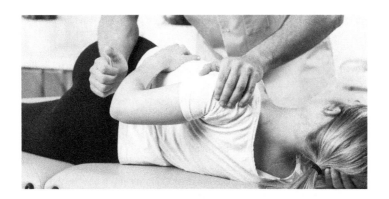

CHIROPRACTIC CARE

Taking care of your spine is like taking care of your car. Every once in a while it needs a tune up! Over the years, trauma, toxins, and thoughts put stress on the spine and nervous system, just as we put miles on a car. Chiropractic care has the incredible ability to meet you where you are on your wellness journey and take your wellness level to the best place it can be through the power of your own body. That is why I fell in love with chiropractic care and began practicing decades ago.

BELOW ARE A FEW REASONS WHY YOU SHOULD INCLUDE CHIROPRACTIC CARE INTO YOUR WELLNESS PLAN

Conservative & Non-Invasive

Chiropractic is a natural, holistic and conservative health care paradigm. It utilizes the body's innate ability to heal itself.

Structural Balance

Chiropractic focuses on the relationship between structure and function. An adjustment can help restore range of motion, keep you flexible and balance proper joint and muscle biomechanics.

Movement = Life To Joints

Movement is essential for the body to work through stress. Chiropractic adjustments help restore movement to joints.

More Focus, More Energy And Improved Sleep

Get out of fight or flight mode. Our bodies are only meant to be stressed for short periods of time, not in a constant state of panic. By balancing the nervous system our organs can get sufficient nerve and blood flow, allowing us to relax muscles, digest and eliminate food properly, breathe deeply and think more clearly.

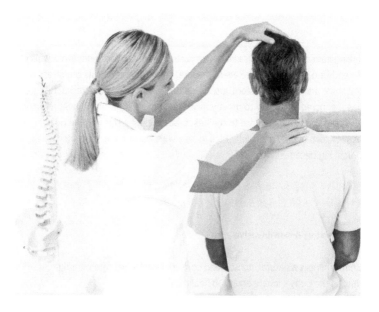

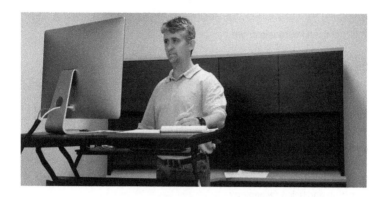

THE POWER OF POSTURE

How's your posture? Did I catch you slouching? As a chiropractor, I see many clients with aches and pains often caused by poor posture. Now, you might be thinking, "Is posture really that important?" Yes, it is.

THE SIDE EFFECTS OF POOR POSTURE

Good posture isn't just about looking better and fitting better in your clothes. It affects how you move and feel.

Poor posture:
- Leads to back pain
- Can lead to digestive problems
- May slow the flow of the lymphatic system
- Reduces lung capacity and can exacerbate asthma
- Can decrease circulation
- Negatively affects sleep
- Has been linked to migraines, neurological problems and depression

"Posture is declining at the speed of technology," shares Dr. Krista Burns with The American Posture Institute.

Dr. Burns, a chiropractor and posture expert, was a competitive skier as a child and young woman. But all those years of sport took a toll on her posture and created severe back pain. After years of seeking solutions she found chiropractic, pain relief and healing. She learned how proper posture and regular adjustments could have prevented her injury and kept her dream alive. Today, Dr. Burns helps young athletes reach peak performance through chiropractic care and posture coaching. Below she shares some tips to undo the damage of poor posture, particularly from the everyday damage caused by sitting and using technology.

UNDOING THE DAMAGE OF SITTING AND TECHNOLOGY

Here are a few simple practices you can incorporate daily to improve posture:

1. Conduct a home posture check. For five minutes, sit up straight at your computer, the top of your monitor positioned at eye level. Keep your knees slightly lower than your hips, and ears directly above your relaxed shoulders. If you find yourself wanting to slouch, you're used to sitting with poor posture.

2. Use earbuds, headphones or a headset when you're on the phone or listening to music.

3. Keep your phone or tablet at eye level when reading, texting, typing or watching anything on it.

4. If you sit in a chair at work that is not ergonomically designed, add a small pillow behind your lower back for lumbar support.

5. Instead of sitting in a chair, try an ergonomic ball for a few hours daily, or consider getting a desk that converts to a standing desk to get you up on your feet.

6. Practice neck retractions. Put your head in a neutral position, facing forward and chin low (not tucked under). Slowly, within a comfortable range of motion, pull your head back over your shoulders.

7. Check your posture regularly and take posture breaks. Every half hour, stand and stretch for 30 seconds. Straighten your arms out, palms up, look up, and squeeze your shoulder blades together. This small action has a greater impact on your postural health than spending 30-minutes at the gym.

8. Do "Wall Angels" daily, particularly in the morning or evening. You can learn how to do them by watching the video linked in the online End Notes, by K's Perfect Fitness. She demonstrates two versions of the exercise. A third version is to move your arms straight up and then back down to the 90 degree angle while keeping arms, back and head against the wall. Do this 5 to 10 times. Watch the video for the basic stance and options for the exercise.

9. Choose a power pose and practice it daily for two minutes. Having good posture is about having a strong body and a strong mind. Research shows that standing tall and proud changes body chemistry. Instead of feeling stressed, people start to feel powerful and in control. Check out social scientist, Amy Cuddy's TED Talk, "Your Body Language Shapes Who You Are," which is linked in the online End Notes.

Maintain good posture by doing these three things consistently:

1. Get regular chiropractic adjustments.

2. Do posture exercises as mentioned above (also check out ideas at www.americanpostureinstitute.com).

3. Change your posture habits using the tips above.

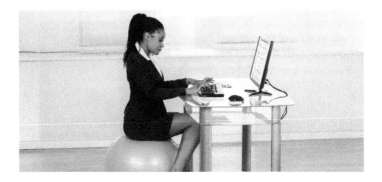

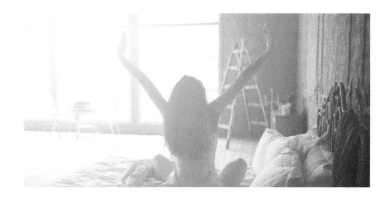

HOW MUCH SLEEP DO YOU NEED?

Adults need 7 to 9 hours of sleep a night. Sleep is essential. There is no substitute for sleep. It is a basic need like water. Our health, productivity, weight, hormone balance, and energy all depend on how we sleep.

GETTING A GOOD NIGHT'S REST

- Reduces anxiety
- Reduces depression
- Stabilizes weight
- Allows your body time to heal
- Reduces signs of aging on your face
- Gives your body an opportunity to detoxify and rejuvenate
- Gives you energy for a full day of activity

HOW TO IMPROVE YOUR SLEEP HABITS

1. Sleep on your side or back with your neck supported in a neutral position (not tilted forward, backward or to either side).

2. Avoid sleeping on your stomach. Stomach sleeping puts a great deal of stress on your neck and lower back.

3. Avoid sleeping with your hands above your head. This cuts off circulation to your arms and hands.

4. Refrain from working on your tablet, cell phone or other electronic device right before going to bed. The light from these devices can trick the brain into thinking that it's daytime and disrupt sleep patterns.

5. Remove the electronics from your bedroom, or if removing them isn't an option, at least don't fall asleep with the TV on. While the noise may distract an overactive mind and help you fall asleep, it will not be conducive to staying asleep. And who knows ... turning off the TV might provide an opportunity to improve your relationship with your partner. Wink, wink. Nudge, nudge.

If you are still having trouble, make an appointment with your family practitioner or doctor.

It's amazing how a number of small changes can radically improve your sleep, so that you're not just catching more zzz's, but getting better quality sleep. In my online program, *21 Days to Rejuvenating Sleep,* I teach you a variety of simple yet powerful tweaks to your sleep habits that make all the difference – everything from sleep posture, to your environment, to night and morning rituals, and mindset shifts. You'll be surprised. You can find it in the Shop on my website at www.drmichellerobin.com.

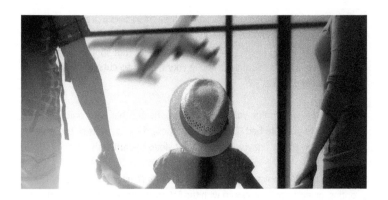

TRAVELING WELL

You can take a few steps before you travel to ensure you feel well on the road. Since you'll have less control over your eating while traveling, try eating "clean" for a few days prior to going on trips.

EATING AND DRINKING ON THE ROAD

Clean eating doesn't have to be complicated. Just try to increase your consumption of vegetables, fruits, beans, raw nuts and seeds, good quality meat protein and non-gluten whole grains (rice, quinoa and millet). You'll also benefit by decreasing your consumption of processed foods, dairy and gluten (wheat, barley, rye, malt and oat-based products).

When traveling, choose protein and veggies as much as possible. If ordering a salad, request the dressing on the side and only use two tablespoons max.

STAY HYDRATED

Breathing dry air can turn you into a blimp by causing you to retain water and swell. Dehydration due to airline air is also a major cause of fatigue. Be sure to drink 8 ounces of water before your flight. More importantly, bring one 16-ounce bottle of water for every 2 hours you'll be in the air, and drink it all before you land. Be sure to consistently drink water (not sports drinks or soda) while you're out and about. It is crucial that you drink water if you are participating in outdoor activities.

PROTECT AGAINST GERMS

If there is ever a time to be sure you frequently wash your hands, it is while you're traveling. Airports, trains, subways, taxis, amusement parks, and meetings with handshaking are ideal places to pick up all sorts of bugs. Hand washing with soap and water is best, but when that's not an option skip the antibacterial gels and instead use essential oils like lemon, clove or thyme. Health food stores also carry alternatives to antibacterial gels.

KEEP YOUR NOSE PRIMED

Hydrate your nose by packing a small 2-ounce bottle of unrefined sesame oil or organic extra virgin olive oil. Dip a cotton swab in the oil and swab around the inside of your nostrils. Pinch your nose. Then breathe in about three times. This gives the nasal passages a barrier to germs and bacteria while also hydrating in dry airplanes and hotel rooms.

PACK SNACKS

Whether you're on a road trip or traveling by air, the options for snacks purchased along the way are mostly unhealthy with inflated prices. Chopped vegetables and fruits, nutrition bars with five or fewer natural ingredients, raw nuts and seeds, and dried fruit can be perfect snacks. They also serve as a quick breakfast on-the-go. Consider fasting on your travel days.

GROCERY SHOP

If I'm going to be somewhere more than a day or two, the first thing I do when I get to town is find a grocery store. I get fresh fruit, veggies, hummus, healthy snack bars, bottled water, and often a big, fresh salad with vinegar and oil on the side. Having these things readily available in the room keeps me from being tempted by the candy machine or room service at the hotel.

It also keeps me stocked with healthy snacks to take with me for each day's outings. If you don't have a mini-fridge in your room you can simply buy only non-perishable items and whole fruit.

KEEP SLEEP SACRED

Set an intentional sleep time. Shut down devices and TV one hour before bed. Pack earplugs and an eye mask to block out distractions. Make sure you're comfortable. If the pillows are too hard or soft ask for something different so that your neck can stay aligned. Use the extra pillows on hotel beds to lie under or between your knees to support your hips and back alignment.

MODIFY YOUR MORNING ROUTINE

If you have a regular morning routine that starts your day off right, don't toss it just because you're traveling. Sure some things won't be the same, but you can anticipate the changes and plan accordingly. For example: bring bags of your favorite morning tea; use an app, like Insight Timer, to give you that meditation bell; pack your workout clothes and find a way to exercise; be sure to have breakfast. If you maintain core elements of your morning routine then you'll start each day strong, as well as make re-entry into post-vacation life easier.

PLAN YOUR WORKOUTS IN ADVANCE

Whether traveling for business or pleasure, it is easy to fully live in the moment and miss out on time to exercise. Schedule your workouts in advance. That way, the time slot will already be filled when you're invited to an impromptu dinner—just politely decline, guilt-free, citing a prior engagement. Make your health a priority so that you have the energy to make the most of your trip.

SUPPLEMENT TO BOOST WELLBEING

Consider traveling with the minimum amount of choice supplements, such as green powder, B vitamins, magnesium, a probiotic, vitamin D and vitamin C. These particular supplements support your immune system, keep your digestive tract healthy and moving, support cellular health and boost your energy.

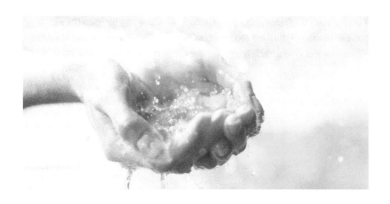

WATER

Adequate hydration is crucial to many of our body's functions, but not all fluids are created equal. Consuming fluid does not necessarily equal hydration. It is important to drink water with nothing added. Flavorings, colors or chemicals in beverages can prevent the water they contain from getting into our cells; and caffeinated beverages and alcohol are actually dehydrating.

TOP HEALTH BENEFITS OF WATER

- Carrying nutrients and oxygen to our cells
- Removing waste products, free radicals and toxins from our cells
- Cushioning bones and lubricating joints
- Regulating body temperature
- Supporting the immune system and digestive processes

Drinking water first thing in the morning (before your coffee or green smoothie) will help get your day off to a great start. It will help replace the water your body lost through respiration and perspiration while you were sleeping, and it will help remove toxins from the nighttime purification process your body has been performing. You might even find that you have more energy.

If you're cold, try drinking hot water with lemon to warm up from the inside out. Be mindful of drinking too much water. If you have a stellar diet then not as much water is required. Too much water can deplete vital nutrients.

Strawberry Mint Infused Water

Ingredients:
2 liters WATER
1 quart fresh STRAWBERRIES
12 MINT LEAVES

Instructions:
Wash all ingredients. Place mint leaves in bottom of pitcher and muddle. Place strawberries in pitcher. Cover with water and let flavors blend overnight.

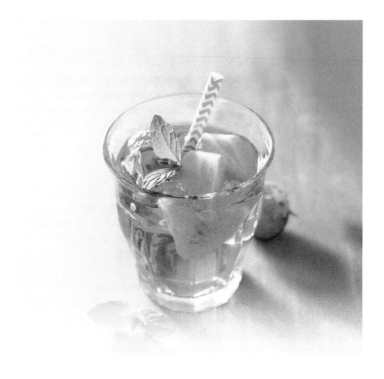

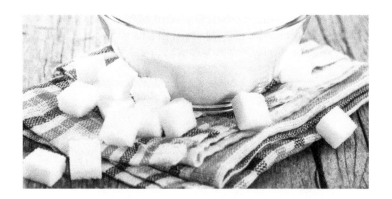

FINDING THE EXTRA SUGAR

Check for hidden sugar in processed foods. It will appear on labels as things like high fructose corn syrup, sucrose, fructose, cane syrup, and cane sugar. And if it's one of the first three ingredients, put the item back on the shelf. You're better off without it. (Note: 4 grams = 1 tsp of sugar.) Added sugar can be found in products like peanut butter, spaghetti sauce, salsas and whole wheat bread.

While it may be tempting to rely on artificial sweeteners to satisfy your sweet tooth, it's not worth the trade-off to your health. Artificial sweeteners can cause a variety of health issues, and despite their low calorie count, they don't help you lose weight. In fact, they have been shown to stimulate the release of insulin, activating your body's storage mode and stimulating your hunger for more sugar.

Sugar consumption increases your body's acidity level, suppresses your immune system, and creates inflammation and an environment for a variety of diseases to thrive, including cancer.

Sugar can cause premature aging. When you consume sugar there is a rapid rise in blood glucose. Your body reacts by secreting insulin to lower the glucose levels. Unfortunately, this suppresses essential hormones and your immune system, both of which help keep you young.

If you feel like you are craving sweets a lot, ask yourself, how else can I treat myself? How else can I add sweetness to my life?

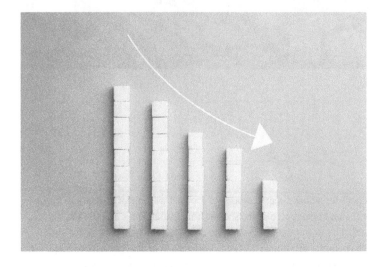

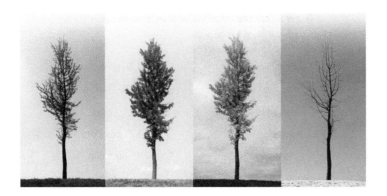

SEASONAL EATING

Our ancestors cultivated their own food from the land and animals. They didn't have processed food, or oranges shipped from the other side of the world in the middle of winter. They ate what was naturally available in each season. Our bodies are actually wired to benefit from the specific foods that grow each season. There are other benefits too, including that what's in season is also at the peak of nutrition, more flavorful, and most affordable. Eating seasonally also supports local farmers and is better for the environment.

GUIDE FOR EATING SEASONALLY

- **In the spring** focus on leafy green vegetables like swiss chard and watercress, also asparagus, avocados, cherries and strawberries.

- **In the summer** focus on light, cooling fruits like berries, peaches and plums. For vegetables try summer squash, cucumber, eggplant, and string beans.

- **In the fall** look for foods that have warming properties and foods that have been harvested like carrots, apples, sweet potatoes, onions, garlic and ginger.

- **In the winter** turn to warming food with higher fat like fish, chicken, beef and lamb. Look for hearty vegetables like kale, collard greens, winter squash, and cabbage.

I've included a list of seasonal vegetables below.

SPRING	SUMMER
Artichokes	Blackberries
Arugula	Blueberries
Asparagus	Corn
Avocados	Cucumbers
Beets	Eggplant
Baby Carrots	Figs
Cauliflower	Melons
Daikon	Nectarines
Dandelion Greens	Okra
Cherries	Peaches
Fava Beans	Peppers
Fennel	Plums
Green Garlic	String Beans
Leeks	Summer Squashes
Mangoes	*(Zucchini, Yellow Crookneck)*
Mixed Baby Greens	Tomatillos
Radishes	Tomatoes
Rhubarb	
Shallots	
Spinach	
Sugar Snap Peas	
Strawberries	
Swiss Chard	
Turnips	
Watercress	

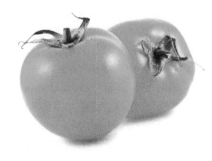

FALL	WINTER
Apples	Bok Choy
Arugula	Cabbage
Asian Pears	Celery Root
Beans	Citrus Fruits
(Cranberry and Shell Beans)	Collard Greens
Bell Peppers	Kale
Broccoli	Leeks
Broccoli Rabe	Parsnips
Brussels Sprouts	Rainbow Chard
Fennel	Rutabagas
Green Tomatoes	Swiss Chard
Hard-shelled Squashes	
(Acorn Squash, Butternut,	
Blue Hubbard, Delicata, Baby	
Dumpling, Pumpkins)	
Pears	
Persimmons	
Pomegranates	
Radicchio	
Sweet Potatoes	

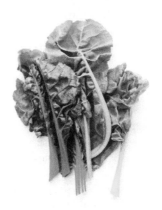

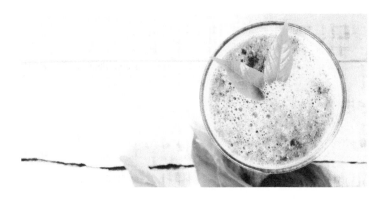

GREEN SMOOTHIES

Depending on the other ingredients you add to your smoothies, they may actually turn out red, purple or brown instead of green. But don't let the color deter you. Even if your eyes don't appreciate it, your insides will definitely thank you for adding dark leafy greens to this delicious morning treat.

TOP HEALTH BENEFITS OF GREEN SMOOTHIES

A stronger immune system: Greens give our cells what they need chemically so that they can function optimally.

Healthier intestinal flora: A healthy gut absorbs nutrients, breeds healthy bacteria and communicates well with the nervous system, keeping the right balance of chemicals in the body.

More balanced blood sugar (fewer spikes and crashes): Greens alkalizing the gut also help regulate the passage of glucose, thus regulating blood sugar.

More energy and better mood: "Higher octane" fuel from nutrient dense foods equals enhanced performance from your body's engine.

Lower risk of cancer: Greens alkalize the body; an overly acidic body is linked to the development of illness and disease, including cancer.

Green smoothies are full of fiber: The fiber in green smoothies helps clean out your colon.

Green Smoothie

Ingredients:
1 cup of WATER or ALMOND MILK
1 – 2 servings of fresh or FROZEN FRUIT
2 handfuls of LEAFY GREENS
1 tbsp organic cold press COCONUT OIL or ½ of a small AVOCADO

Instructions:
Put all ingredients in blender. Blend until smooth.

Greens have oxalic acid, it is important to rotate greens.
*** If you are on a blood thinner be mindful how many leafy greens you are using.*

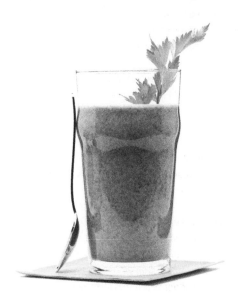

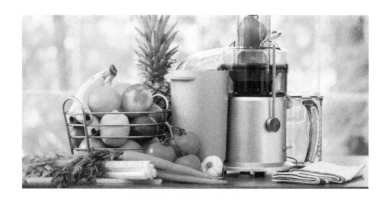

JUICE

If green smoothies aren't your thing, or you're looking for an alternative to smoothies when the weather turns chillier, consider juicing. You might even try juicing as a great mid-afternoon snack. When juicing vegetables, there is no need to peel anything as long as your produce is organic. If your produce isn't organic you need to peel. You can learn more about juicing by listening to my interview with Steve Spangler, former pro-athlete and owner of Simple Science Juices. The link to the podcast is in the online End Notes.

TOP BENEFITS OF JUICING

Easily digested: Your body doesn't have to put as much energy into breaking down your food, and the nutrients are more readily absorbed into your system.

Boosts the nutritional value of your meal: Juicing provides a plethora of nutrients and minerals, and you'll get the health benefits of far more fruits and vegetables than you'd actually be able to eat.

Improves heart health: Juicing vegetables increases the amount of powerful antioxidants in your blood and lowers triglyceride levels. And as an added bonus, you might lose a few extra pounds, reducing the strain on your heart.

Naturally provides beneficial enzymes and phytochemicals: Found primarily in raw food, the enzymes in fresh fruits and vegetables convert food into body tissue and energy, and phytochemicals are powerful disease fighters.

Helps repair and rejuvenate the body: Because it's loaded with so many vitamins, minerals and other phytochemicals, it provides your body with the tools it needs to repair and rejuvenate itself; and because it's naturally gluten and dairy-free, your body has less to assimilate.

Pineapple Juice Blend

Ingredients:
1/4 PINEAPPLE
2-4 stalks CELERY
1/2 CUCUMBER
1/2 LEMON
1 handful CILANTRO
tiny piece GINGER

Instructions:
Wash all ingredients. Push all ingredients one at a time through your juicer.
Then serve and enjoy!

Use very little if any fruit because it can cause an insulin spike.

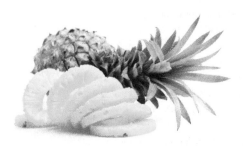

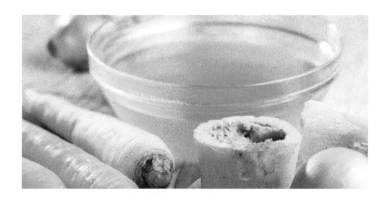

BONE BROTH

You probably have been hearing about bone broth a lot lately. It has some pretty amazing benefits. Bone broth helped me on my own healing journey too. Shelly Murray, my health coach, started her own Bone Broth business, The Broth Pot. If you are in Missouri or Kansas and want a rich, clean Bone Broth you'll find Shelly's contact information on the online End Notes web page.

TOP HEATH BENEFITS OF BONE BROTH

- Helps heal and seal your gut and promotes healthy digestion
- Reduces joint pain and inflammation
- Promotes strong healthy bones
- Inhibits infection
- Fights inflammation
- Promotes healthy hair and nail growth

HOW TO INCORPORATE BONE BROTH

- Drink ½ cup first thing in the morning
- Drink ½ cup with lunch and dinner

- Use bone broth to make soups
- Use bone broth in other recipes that call for liquid (taco meat, any whole grain dish)

Chicken Bone Broth

Ingredients:
4 lb CHICKEN bones, FEET, GIBBLETS, LIVER, NECK
Filtered Cold Water
2 TBL APPLE CIDER VINEGAR
BONES from the cooked CHICKEN
1 large yellow ONION, quartered
2-4 CELERY, with leaves
2-4 CARROTS
2-3 PARSNIPS
1-2 TURNIPS
2 tsp SEA SALT
1 strip KOMBU

Instructions:
Put your chicken bones, feet, neck, gizzards, heart and liver into a large stock pot. Cover the chicken with cold filtered water. The water should be 1 inch above the bones. Add 2 TBL APPLE CIDER VINEGAR and let set 1 hour. Turn heat to high and allow the water to come to a boil. Turn the heat down so that the water is barely simmering. Cover with lid. After a few hours of cooking add in ONION, CELERY, CARROTS, PARSNIPS, TURNIPS, SEA SALT and KOMBU. You may have to add in more water.

Cover with a lid. Check the broth periodically to make sure it is simmering at the proper temperature. Continue to cook the broth for up to 24-48 hours. A longer cooking time makes more flavorful broth and extracts more nutrition from the bones. Turn off the heat and allow your broth to cool a bit, then strain it into another pot to remove BONES and VEGETABLES. Pour the broth into heat-safe containers and store in the fridge or freezer. Warm up broth and sip on like coffee or tea or turn your broth into your favorite soup or stew.

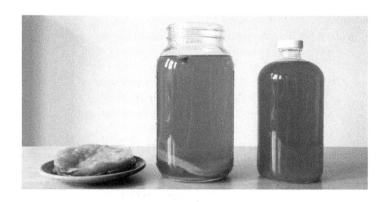

FERMENTED FOODS

Fermented foods might sound odd, but I bet you've had them before, whether you knew they were fermented or not. There are many important benefits to adding fermented foods into your diet, including: natural probiotics / good gut bacteria, important nutrients, optimizing your immune system, detoxification, and a healthy variety of microflora.

HOW TO INCORPORATE FERMENTED FOODS

First, figure out which fermented foods you like. Start out slowly. You may want to begin by trying 1-2 TBL of fermented foods with lunch and dinner. You could do 4 oz of Kombucha or 1/2 cup of Beet Kvass into your daily meal plan.

FERMENTED FOODS

- Tempeh
- Miso
- Yogurt (Plain)
- Kefir (Homemade)
- Beet Kvass
- Kombucha

- Sauerkraut
- Kimchi
- Chutneys

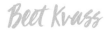

Beet Kvass

Ingredients:
2 large BEETS, peeled and coarsely chopped
1/8 cup homemade WHEY
(from strained homemade yogurt or sauerkraut juice)
2 tsp - 1/2 TBL SEA SALT
Filtered WATER

Instructions:
Place BEETS, WHEY and SEA SALT in a 1 quart mason jar. Add filtered WATER to fill the container and stir well. Keep at room temperature for 2-3 days on your countertop. Store in the door of your refrigerator. To serve pour through a strainer. Save some of the liquid before starting a new batch and use the liquid instead of the WHEY for the next batch.

Note: 1/4 cup in the morning and evening is an excellent blood tonic. It promotes regularity, aids digestion, alkalizes the blood, cleanses the liver, and is a good treatment for kidney stones.

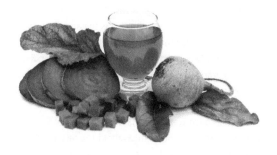

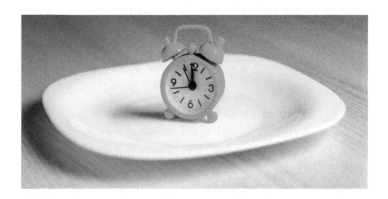

INTERMITTENT FASTING

Intermittent fasting is the practice of making a conscious decision of when to eat and when to skip certain meals. People practice intermittent fasting in a number of ways.

- Some people choose to eat only from 11:00am to 7:00pm. Essentially they skip breakfast and then consume all their calories in an 8-hour window.
- Others choose to skip two meals in a day and take a full 24-hours off from eating. To do this they eat on a normal schedule and finish their last meal at 3:00pm. Then the next day they don't eat anything again until 3:00pm.
- A 13-hour fast is a great option for many and can be done daily. You simply end your last meal by 7:00pm and consume only water or herbal tea from then until 8:00am.

No matter which approach you take to fasting it is critical that you drink half your bodyweight in ounces in water throughout the fast. (150lbs = 75 oz of water) Staying hydrated is important for your body to function properly, to keep you from getting headaches, to keep your energy up during the fast, and to help flush out toxins.

I've been experimenting with different fasts myself and try to fast once a week. It feels like a mini reset for my body and mind.

Now you might be thinking, why in the world would anyone in their right mind do this to themselves? What are the benefits? Isn't breakfast good for you? Is it dangerous?

Fasting is definitely not a new concept. Fasting has been a practice in many cultures and religions throughout history. As early as the 1930s, scientists have been exploring the benefits of fasting, and it is an even more popular research topic in the scientific community today.

Here are just some benefits to intermittent fasting that are being found through research:

- It can slow down the aging process
- It can help with weight loss
- It can normalize insulin sensitivity
- It can help prevent cancer and other diseases
- It can improve your eating patterns
- It can improve memory and clear-thinking

If you're new to fasting you can take baby steps. Before you start a more dramatic fast try using bone broth instead of fully skipping a meal. Bone Broth is incredibly nutritious and the protein will help sustain you throughout your fast.

Disclaimer: Always consult a doctor before fasting or making a drastic lifestyle or diet change, especially if you have a chronic health condition.

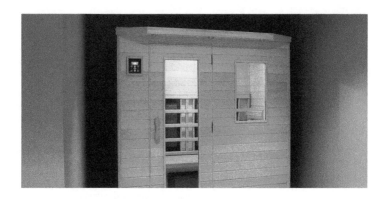

3-IN-1 INFRARED THERAPY

3-in-1 infrared therapy is a type of sauna therapy from Sunlighten™ that combines near, mid and far infrared energy to assist with detoxification, relaxation, lower blood pressure, weight loss, pain relief, anti-aging and energize from the inside out.

Sunlighten™ 3-in-1 saunas can be found at wellness centers around the globe or can be easily installed in your home! You can learn more about infrared therapy by listening to my interview with Connie Zach of Sunlighten™. The link to the podcast is in the online End Notes.

TOP BENEFITS OF 3-IN-1 THERAPY

Purify. Sweating is the natural and safe way for the body to heal and stay healthy. Sweat carries toxins out of the body and pushes them through the pores. Far infrared (FIR) has the ability to heat the body directly, increasing core body temperature resulting in a deep sweat at the cellular level where toxins reside. Other FIR benefits include weight loss, blood pressure reduction and relaxation.

Slenderize. Studies have shown that benefits of mid infrared (MIR) energy can burn calories while you relax. As the body works to cool itself, there is a substantial increase in heart rate, cardiac output and metabolic rate, causing the body to burn more calories. A study using Sunlighten™ saunas showed a reduction in weight and waist circumference in just a three month period with regular use. Other MIR benefits include pain relief and improved circulation.

Energize. Near infrared (NIR) energy can help strengthen the immune system and boost energy. In fact, a NASA study showed near infrared therapy, delivered by LEDs deep into body tissue, can quadruple cell health and tissue growth. Several studies have shown that LEDs stimulate white blood cell production and collagen growth by increasing energy at the cellular level. Other NIR benefits include cell health, wound healing, pain relief and anti-aging.

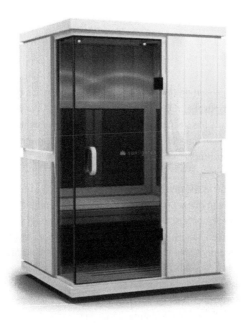

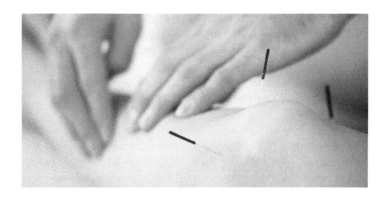

ACUPUNCTURE CARE

ACUPUNCTURE 101: WHAT YOU NEED TO KNOW

It seems odd that inserting tiny needles into various points on our body can be healing, but for over 5,000 years, as part of Traditional Chinese Medicine (TCM), acupuncture has been used to effectively treat a wide range of health conditions. It is recommended by the World Health Organization as a safe and beneficial wellness modality.

TCM views disease as the result of an imbalance, deficiency, or blockage in the body's natural energy flow. Such imbalances manifest in physical, emotional, and stress-related disorders. The TCM approach is focused on strengthening the body rather than merely treating symptoms. It is about preventative medicine that prolongs life rather than reactive medicine that prevents death.

Acupuncture is a method of balancing and building the body's life force energy known as "qi" or "chi" so the body can heal itself. This energy follows the same laws and principles of nature within your body.

Your body consists of 12 major energy channels or meridians. These meridians are responsible for 'transporting' life energy throughout your body. They influence the nervous system, muscles, organs, and hormones.

If your are experiencing energy blockages in one of your meridians, you can feel both emotional and physical pain.

Depending on where your energy block is occurring you might struggle with anxiety, depression, lack of energy, digestion issues, inflammation issues, lack of appetite, brain fog, hot flashes, hormone imbalances, irritability, joint pain, chronic pain, sleep issues, or any other common symptoms. Acupuncture has also been used to support those suffering from PTSD.

Our energy and its ability to flow through our body unobstructed affects how we feel, how we think, and our overall health.

WHAT YOU CAN EXPECT

You will sit or lie down. The acupuncturist will gently insert tiny disposable needles along the meridians to stimulate and unblock energy flow. For most people the needles don't cause any pain or discomfort. Once the needles are inserted, you'll relax, on average, for 30 minutes. Everyone has a unique experience, but many people are so deeply relaxed that they fall asleep during the session.

This 30 minute session of energy work has the ability to increase blood flow, brain chemistry, and release pain-reducing hormones. Women struggling with infertility have been known to become pregnant after acupuncture therapy sessions. People suffering from chronic migraines, depression, urinary tract infections, fatigue or arthritis have been known to feel relief even after a single acupuncture session.

Go to the Acupuncture section of the online End Notes web page for links to videos and contact information to learn more

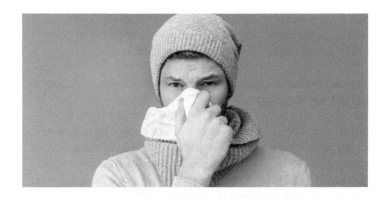

SURVIVING ALLERGY, COLD & FLU SEASON

There's just no getting around it: Once the temperature drops, the return of cold season reliably comes with it. The annual threat of the flu is always close behind. Allergies are more likely to happen year round depending on the person.

HERE ARE A FEW TIPS TO HELP YOU SURVIVE AND THRIVE THROUGH ALLERGIES AND THE COLD AND FLU SEASON

- Go dairy-free during Allergy Season. Dairy is very mucus forming
- Try oil pulling. It is easy. Take a tablespoon of organic coconut oil or unrefined sesame oil into your mouth and swish for 5-20 minutes. Do not swallow. Spit the oil out in a lined trash can
- Scrape your tongue, using a tongue scraper you get at the drugstore
- Brush and floss your teeth twice daily
- Stay hydrated
- Use the Nasopure Nasal Wash System or the Neti Pot during allergy season

- Rehydrate your nasal passages with EVOO (extra virgin olive oil) or unrefined sesame oil. Use a Q-tip dipped in the oil and rim the inside of your nostril, then breath in by pinching your nose. This provides an extra barrier against germs and allergens
- Eat a diet high in vegetables, especially cooked leafy greens, berries and green tea
- When temperatures drop and the wind kicks up, keep your neck covered. This will help hold your body heat in and keep the chill at bay
- Wash your hands
- If you feel like you're coming down with something, eat a very simple diet of steamed vegetables, bone broths, vegetable soups and/or vegetable juices
- At the first sign of sickness, drop into Whole Foods or check out the online Thrive Market or another natural food store and pick up a bottle of Elderberry concentrate. Take one tablespoon three times a day

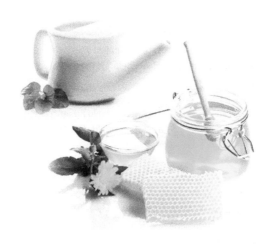

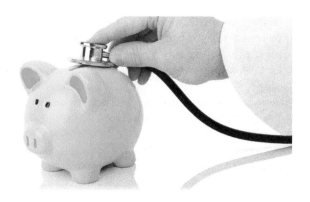

YOUR FINANCIAL WELLBEING

Money may not buy happiness, but financial wellbeing is an important part of overall wellness. Why? Financial stress impacts your health physically and emotionally. Building your financial wellbeing is part of "crediting" your health account.

Look to a financial advisor for specific wealth building advice and read below for mindset and management ideas that will build your financial wellbeing.

OPEN YOUR MAIL

If you're nervous about money or feel like it is over your head you may avoid dealing with it. Soon you have stacks of mail that become overwhelming. Start taking control of your money by opening it. Awareness is the first step.

INVEST IN YOUR HEALTH

If you've accumulated wealth while letting your health degrade then you've lost your greatest asset. Choose to invest in your wellness now so that you can enjoy your wealth in both finances and health later.

VALUE EXPERIENCES OVER STUFF

Collect memories instead of things. If you spend money on experiences they last a lifetime, consistently giving you joy and connection to others. That's a lot better than the limited warranty of most stuff.

RESPECT YOUR MONEY

Keep your cash nicely organized in an uncluttered wallet. Keep your financial records organized and your checkbook balanced.

BUY WISELY

If you're making a big purchase, sleep on it to avoid buyer's remorse and impulsive decisions.

CREATE A REALISTIC BUDGET AND USE IT

Create buckets of money for living expenses, fun, emergency fund, savings, charity, health, and investments. Keep track of your income and expenses. Review budgeted versus actual numbers quarterly, at a minimum.

BE GENEROUS

Give to your favorite non-profits and/or faith community. Also donate your time and talents by volunteering.

SAVE FOR THE FUTURE

Contribute to your retirement accounts, other investments, or savings. Make this an automatic process so that you aren't tempted to use that money elsewhere.

MANAGE YOUR CREDIT

Credit cards can be helpful if used and managed correctly. Be mindful of the number of cards you have, the limits, and interest rates. Payoff your balance monthly and timely.

TEACH YOUR CHILDREN THE VALUE OF MONEY

Give your children lessons on what money is, its different forms, and how it is saved and used. Give them the opportunity to earn, save and spend their own money even when they're little. As they're older have frank conversations about money.

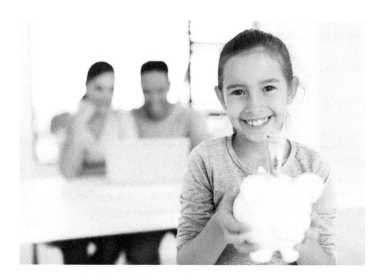

YOUR NEXT SMALL CHANGES

I'm so grateful that you've taken the time to read this short book. I hope you've gleaned a few new nuggets of wisdom and fresh ideas. Perhaps you're even seeing your wellness journey and the possibilities of improved wellbeing in a new light, doable, and with greater hope. That's my wish for you.

The subtitle of this book, and an earlier section, is "Put the Odds in Your Favor." There's a reason for that. Every effort, every change you make, no matter how small, credits your wellness account. You're building health and resilience. You're growing and strengthening the roots of your wellbeing. That's true no matter where you stand currently on the wellbeing spectrum. Trust in your journey and take the next step, and then the next.

YOUR FIRST NEXT STEP

Start with gratitude. It's easy to chastise and shame our bodies, to point out everything that's "wrong." Consider making your next step on your wellness journey one of gratitude. Be grateful for the body you currently have. Your body is doing the best it can right now to care for you.

In the next section there is space for you to celebrate everything good about your body, mind, and spirit. Take the time to celebrate all that you are and all that your body does for you. As an example, I'm grateful that I was able to swim this morning and move my body, that I had the strength, control, flexibility and stamina to be able to take care of chiropractic clients this afternoon, and that I can see the smiles and hear the laughter of my family when I get home tonight.

I encourage you to keep a gratitude journal for everything in your life. But also, remember to be grateful for your body each and every day.

This book is filled with many tips for creating your wellness plan. Some of them probably spoke to you while others may not have at this time. We're all different in what we like, what we need, and what we're capable of doing right now.

Go back to the section of this book where I outline the Quadrants of Wellbeing. Also, consider watching the videos about the quadrants at www.quadrantsofwellbeing.com. The Quadrants of Wellbeing is a framework for viewing your whole being wellness.

On the following pages you'll see a page with the icon for the Quadrants of Wellbeing. Each quadrant is labeled with a brief description. Use the space provided to identify just a few small changes you'd like to incorporate into your healthy habits.

Often our behavior pattern is to take on a lot of change at once or take drastic measures. Instead, select one, just one small change you're going to focus on right now. Do that one, simple change consistently for at least a month before you add in another good habit. Take that time to notice how that one small change has likely created a bigger shift in your wellbeing than you expected. Also, notice how you may have made the change to impact one particular quadrant, but it has actually shifted your wellbeing in other quadrants as well. Funny how that works.

Keep on moving forward in your wellness journey. Inch by inch, wellness is a cinch! Refer back to this book or my other books, blogs, podcast, or the resources listed in the back, or on the End Notes web page, as you keep adding new small changes and healthy habits into your life.

Wishing you love and hugs,

Michelle Robin

I'M GRATEFUL FOR AND CELEBRATE

Use the space below to celebrate everything good about your body, mind, and spirit. Take the time to celebrate all that you are and all that your body does for you.

MY QUADRANTS OF WELLBEING PLAN

Use the space below to identify a few small changes you'll make in the coming months/years for each quadrant. Write them in the space provided for each quadrant. Remember to keep it simple. Add only one or two small changes into your life at a time. Focus on fully integrating a small change before you start working on another one. Keep it simple and consistent to avoid overwhelm and to increase your chances of lasting change. Trust me that making even one small change will create big shifts in your wellbeing.

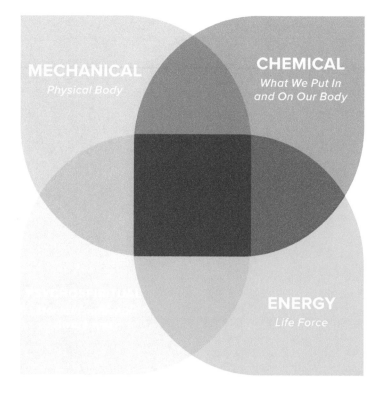

MECHANICAL:

CHEMICAL:

ENERGY:

PSYCHOSPIRITUAL:

WAYS I'VE IMPROVED MY WELLNESS

On any journey, it's important to acknowledge how far you've come. Your wellness journey is no different. I encourage you to take a moment to jot down and celebrate your successes.

POWERED BY the Y

I am honored to have YMCA of Greater Kansas City as a partner this year. I reached out to the Y because I believe in their mission and three pillars - youth development, healthy living, and social responsibility. They are a robust resource throughout our community and across the nation. As much as they are helping us spread the message of Small Changes Big Shifts,℠ I want to shine a spotlight on all the good they do, and how you may want to include the Y as a resource for your wellness journey.

In this anniversary year I'm focused on four words: celebrate, guide, connect, and how they lead to hope. The Y is part of creating hope, for individuals, families and communities by...

- **Celebrating** and welcoming the rich diversity - in every lovely expression of that word - in our communities; and cheering on their members' successes along the way
- **Guiding** members in their wellness journeys regardless of fitness level, needs, or age; offering a wide variety of fitness opportunities, educational, wellness, and social programs
- **Connecting** individuals and families with one another; acting as a central hub for not only wellness resources, and individual wellbeing, but social connection as well

When people feel welcomed and celebrated, when they know they have a resource to help guide them in innumerable ways, when they feel a sense of connection and belonging, they have hope. That hope may energize their day. It may be the extra push they need to move through difficult times in their life. That hope may be what reminds them that they are loved and a valuable part of the community. We all need this and the Y delivers.

I encourage you to look into ways that the Y in your community may have services or programs that would support your needs.

- 14 Y locations throughout the metro, all with full fitness centers and 12 with pools
- 90+ Before and after school program locations throughout the metro
- 12+ Early learning and Head Start programs to prepare children for success in school
- 20+ Summer Day Camps throughout the metro
- Nutrition, personal training and weight loss
- Group exercise classes, adult sports and group interest programs to help you stay active and make connections
- Education and lifestyle change for chronic disease prevention and management
- Exercise and social activities for older adults, 55+
- Swim lessons and water safety to provide life-saving skills to all ages
- Youth sports for ages as young as 3, plus youth swim clubs and teams
- Adaptive sports and social programs for youth and young adults with physical, developmental and intellectual disabilities
- Kid Zone where the kids can have fun while you work out
- Family events and activities for quality time together
- Youth leadership and enrichment
- Volunteer opportunities for youth and adults

Learn more about locations, specific programs, facilities, and membership at www.kansascityymca.org. If you live outside the KC metro area look for a Y near you by visiting www.ymca.net.

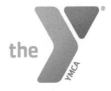

YMCA OF GREATER KANSAS CITY

RECOMMENDED RESOURCES

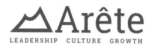

Arête
www.arete-hpa.com

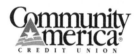

Community America
www.communityamerica.com

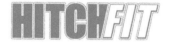

Hitch Fit
www.hitchfit.com

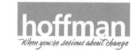

Hoffman Institute Foundation
www.hoffmaninstitute.org

INDIGO WILD

Indigo Wild
www.indigowild.com

notes to self.
words make all the difference

Notes to Self

www.notestoself.com

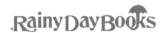

Rainy Day Books

www.rainydaybooks.com

Simple Science Juices

www.simplesciencejuices.com

State Line
Animal Hospital
&
Holistic Health
913-381-3272 | statelineah.com

State Line Animal Hospital & Holistic Health

www.statelineah.com

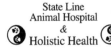 sunlighten™

Sunlighten

www.sunlighten.com

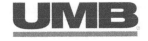

UMB

www.umb.com

RECOMMENDED READING

Below are my favorite books on a variety of health and wellbeing topics. I've also listed them in the online End Notes where you can just click a link to buy on Amazon, for your convenience.

The E Factor: Engage, Energize, Enrich —Three Steps to Vibrant Health by Dr. Michelle Robin

Wellness on a Shoestring: Seven Habits for a Healthy Life by Dr. Michelle Robin

The Autoimmune Solution by Amy Myers

Rising Strong by Brené Brown

The Whole30: The 30-Day Guide to Total Health and Food Freedom Book by Dallas Hartwig and Melissa Hartwig

The Blender Girl Smoothies: 100 Gluten-Free, Vegan, and Paleo-Friendly Recipes by Tess Masters

The Reboot with Joe Juice Diet: Lose Weight, Get Healthy and Feel Amazing by Joe Cross

Breaking Night: A Memoir of Forgiveness, Survival, and My Journey from Homeless to Harvard by Liz Murray

On Fire: The 7 Choices to Ignite a Radically Inspired Life by John O'Leary

No Sweat: How the Simple Science of Motivation Can Bring You a Lifetime of Fitness by Michelle Segar

Uplifting Prayers to Light Your Way: 200 Invocations for Challenging Times by Sonia Choquette

The Natural Pregnancy Book by Aviva Jill Romm and Ina May Gaskin

The Oz Family Kitchen: More Than 100 Simple and Delicious Real Food Recipes from Our Home to Yours by Lisa Oz and Mehmet Oz M.D.

Effortless Healing: 9 Simple Ways to Sidestep Illness, Shed Excess Weight, and Help Your Body Fix Itself by Dr. Joseph Mercola and David Perlmutter M.D.

This Is Your Do-Over: The 7 Secrets to Losing Weight, Living Longer, and Getting a Second Chance at the Life You... by Michael F. Roizen and Mehmet Oz

The Power of Self-Healing: Unlock Your Natural Healing Potential in 21 Days by Fabrizio Mancini

Brain Maker: The Power of Gut Microbes to Heal and Protect Your Brain–for Life by David Perlmutter and Kristin Loberg

May I Be Frank: How I Changed My Ways, Lost 100 Pounds, and Found Love Again by Frank Ferrante and Marianne Williamson

Wheat Belly Total Health: The Ultimate Grain-Free Health & Weight-Loss Life Plan by William Davis

The Wahls Protocol: A Radical New Way to Treat All Chronic Autoimmune Conditions Using Paleo Principles by Terry Wahls M.D. and Eve Adamson

The Mayo Clinic Handbook for Happiness: A Four-Step Plan for Resilient Living by Amit Sood MD and Mayo Clinic

I Declare: 31 Promises to Speak Over Your Life by Joel Osteen

The Self-Compassion Diet: A Step-by-Step Program to Lose Weight with Loving-Kindness by Jean Fain

Same Kind of Different As Me: A Modern-Day Slave, an International Art Dealer, and the Unlikely Woman Who Bound Them Together by Ron Hall, Denver Moore and Lynn Vincent

Ask Dr. Nandi: 5 Steps to Becoming Your Own #HealthHero™ for Longevity, Well-Being, and a Joyful Life by Dr. Partha Nandi

Dr. Michelle Robin℠

ADDRESS	7410 Switzer, Shawnee Mission, KS 66203
PHONE	(913) 962-7408
WEBSITE	www.DrMichelleRobin.com
EMAIL	mRobin@DrMichelleRobin.com
FACEBOOK	www.facebook.com/drmichellerobin
TWITTER	www.twitter.com/drmichellerobin

AVAILABLE FOR PURCHASE

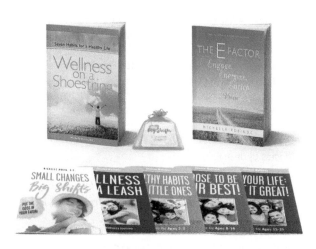

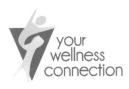

your
wellness
connection

a wellness partnership™

ADDRESS	7410 Switzer, Shawnee Mission, KS 66203
PHONE	(913) 962-7408
WEBSITE	www.YourWellnessConnection.com
EMAIL	info@YourWellnessConnection.com
FACEBOOK	www.facebook.com/yourwellnessconnection
TWITTER	www.twitter.com/wellness_kc

YOUR WELLNESS CONNECTION

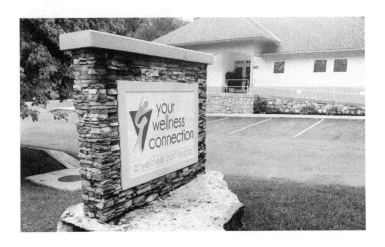

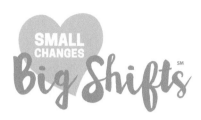

The Small Changes Big Shifts podcast is your weekly dose of wellness encouragement. It's the small changes that stick and ultimately compound to create big shifts in our holistic wellbeing. Renowned guests will share wisdom, knowledge, real life stories and practical tips to inspire and inform you as you move forward on your journey to a life of wellness.

SMALL CHANGES BIG SHIFTS PODCAST
www.drmichellerobin.com/small-changes-big-shifts

 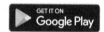

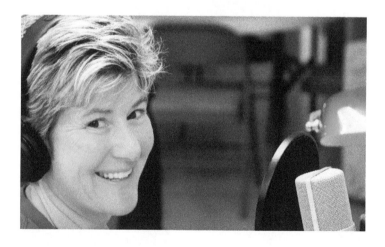